I0415266

BEST DETOX DIETS

Detoxification Book with Step By Step weight Loss Cleanse

Powerful Detox Diets for Releasing Weight, Increase Energy and Rejuvenating the body

Amy D Morse

Published by Amy D Morse, 2019

While every Precaution has been taken in the preparation of this book, the Publisher assumes no responsibility for errors or omissions, or damages resulting from the use of the information contained herein.

BEST DETOX DIETS

Detoxification Book with Step By Step weight Loss Cleanse

First edition. March 12, 2019.

Copyright © 2019 Amy D Morse

Written by Amy D Morse

LEGAL DISCLAIMER

The information in this eBook is not intended to replace medical advice.

No action or inaction should be taken based solely on the contents of this information.

Before beginning this or any other nutritional or exercise regimen, consult your physician to be sure it is appropriate for you.

The information and opinions expressed here are believed to be accurate, based on the best judgement of this author.

Readers who fail to consult with appropriate health authorities assume the risk of any injuries.

ALL RIGHTS RESERVED.

This eBook contains material protected under International and Federal Copyright Laws and Treaties. Any unauthorized reprint or use of this material is prohibited. No part of this eBook may be reproduced or transmitted in any form or by any means, electronic or mechanical, including photocopying, recording, or by any information storage and retrieval system without express written permission from the author.

Tables of Contents

ATTENTION: GET YOUR FREE GIFTS

Download 4 of the best weight loss eBooks absolutely for free. These eBooks will help you Detox, Cleanse your body system and shed excess body weight, get rid of stubborn belly fat and get body shape of your dream.

Click the Pictures Below to Download

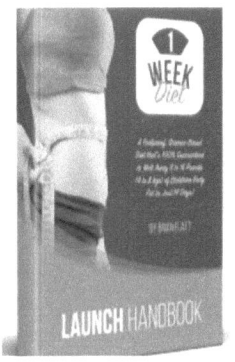 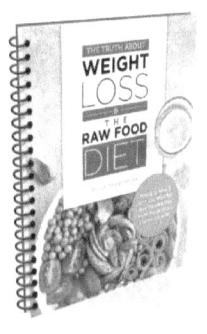

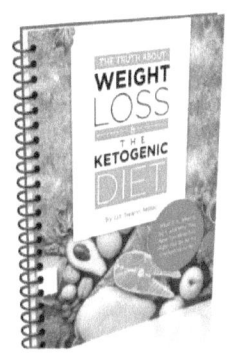 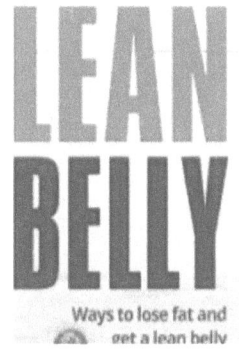

If Truly, You enjoy reading this eBook, kindly **leave your honest review** at the end.

The end.

Thank You.

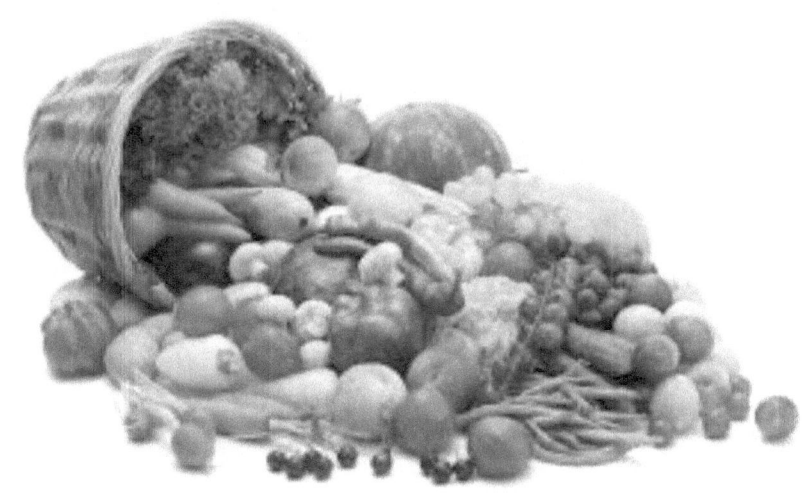

Introduction to Detox Diet for Weight loss

Detox Diets are the best for body cleansing. You can detox regularly by using the detox diet plan as a regular part of your lifestyle. Proper detox diet will make you lose weight and feel lighter and better than ever before.

You may have heard about toxins, detoxification, cleansing, purifying they are all related to detox diets.

Toxins are harmful chemicals affecting your body. They are all around you (in your food, water, air) and inside you (as waste products of metabolism).

Your body eliminates most toxins and the rest are stored within body fat.

These stored toxins combined with stress can affect your health in an unpleasant ways:

- Weight gain

- Headaches

- Feelings of fatigue and weakness

- Heartburn

- Sore muscles and skin

- Joint pains

These symptoms will fade when you embark on total body detox.

Well, you may feel some discomfort in the very first days, but that is a normal body reaction.

You may feel a headache or sore muscle that is because the toxins are released faster than your body can eliminate them.

These symptoms will not occur again if you detox regularly.

Body that is overloaded with toxins cannot perform its normal cleansing job that is required for optimal health. In addition to naturally-occurring toxins, it is estimated that more than 400 man-made chemicals as well as heavy metals permeate the body of a person on a daily basis. Naturally if these toxins are not removed from the body, they can cause chronic health ailments. It is therefore very necessary to Detox and cleanse the body from these toxins and pollutants.

Detox diet plan involves Taking necessary actions regarding every area of your health (Colon, lungs, bowel, liver, skin etc) simply because toxins overload will create a wide range of symptoms and conditions--and transform your health in ways you've never imagined. An important step in a full body detox is to restore and replenish energy levels to make you more alert in different areas of your life, such as at work. Body detox is a great way to give your body a boost after a night of over-indulgence, eating all the wrong foods and consuming more alcohol than is healthy. That is why body Detox is needed because some mortals are having this kind of lifestyle.

What if you could focus on your body aspect of your well-being to transform all the others--and at the same time prevent health problems you didn't even know were lurking beneath the surface? In today's world, we have no idea how many symptoms, conditions, and diseases are rooted in an overloaded liver. It's not only about liver cancer, cirrhosis, and hepatitis. Nearly every challenge--from pesky general health complaints to digestive issues to emotional struggles to weight gain to high blood pressure to heart problems to brain fog to skin conditions to autoimmune and other chronic illnesses--has an origin in an overloaded liver and can improve and heal when you harness the force of this humble organ. Detox diet plan offers the answers you should have had all along. Amy d Morse shares unparalleled insights into undiscovered functions of our life-saving organs, explains what's behind dozens of health issues that hold us back, and offers detailed guidance on how to move forward so we can live our best lives. Find out for yourself what detox diet plan is all about: being clearer-headed, more peaceful, happier, and better able to adapt to our fast-changing times. Learn how to sleep well, balance blood sugar, lower blood pressure, lose weight, and look and feel younger. A healthy body organ (liver, colon, lungs etc) is the ultimate de-stressor, anti-aging ally, and safeguard against a threatening world--if we give it the right support. The path to a healthy body and happy belly is paved with real food—fresh, wholesome, sustainable food—and it doesn't need to be so difficult.

An internal body cleansing can have many great benefits. Cleansing your body of toxic build up can provide relief from fatigue, tension, headaches, constipation, skin problems and acne and PMS, just to name a few.

Click here to start detox-Cleansing Now

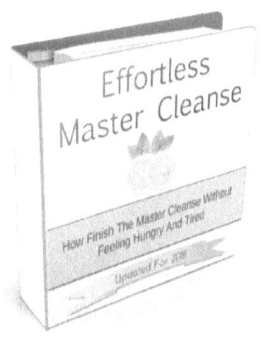

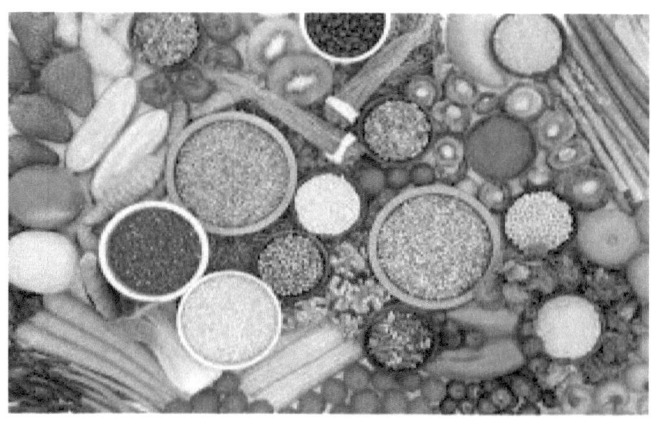

How to Detox Your Body

Most popular body cleansing detoxification processes is fasting, People fast to clean up the accumulated Toxins and harmful substances away from the body. Fasting can be done either with only water or varieties of juices. Although food is very important in supplying the body nutrients for energy and body processes, sometimes the body uses too much energy digesting foods and less time purging toxins out of the body. If you are familiar with body detoxing through fasting, you can jump-start your body organs to begin the cleansing process so as to eliminate all the toxic build-up from your system.

Fasting Procedure

For so many years People had been fasting to cleanse the body of Toxins. You too can embark on fasting to detox your body.

The great question to ask is why the body better detoxifies itself during a period of fasting. You expect that you might grow weak without proper nourishment for several days during fasting period but just think about all the energy your body uses during the digestive process … there is no energy left over for cleansing the body.

How to detox your body should start with fasting because it has proven to be a successful way to cleanse yourself from the inside out. Because when you are not eating food and just drinking water (or juice), your body expends its energy focusing on the different eliminating body organs like the liver, kidneys, intestines and skin.

Same applies to when you are sick - you usually do not feel like eating and not have the urge even though your stomach rumbles. This same principle applies here on how to detox your body. The cleansing process is considered to be the illness your body must defend itself against – thus cleansing itself of harmful toxins.

Types of Fasting

There are different types of fasting to solve the problem of how to detox your body.

Complete water fast where you drink just water throughout your length of fasting.

You can learn how to detox your body through juice fasts

or what is called a mono food fast.

To start a juice fast, you must create your very own fresh juices each day and don't buy from store, unless you are sure is all natural and fresh, must be through an organic whole foods store. Body detox through juice fasting is likely more attractive and palatable than the pure form. The rule for juice fasting is to choose only one fruit or vegetable that has cleansing properties e.g. carrots, watermelons or any fruits with

antioxidants. This will
supply the body with the fuel
it needs without exhausting
the digestive system.

Monofood fasting

**This is another option to
detox your body and it
involves eating only one type
of food** — either one
vegetable or fruit — that has
cleansing and antioxidant
properties. It works the same
way as juice fasting you can
select only one vegetable or
fruit, combinations of fruits
are not allowed.

To detox your body can be quite easy, but it required some effort to stay true to course because you will become very hungry and want to eat. Therefore, if you can stick to the plan for just two or three days, figuring out how to detox your body will become a whole lot easier.

Repeat the process once or twice a year will be sufficient and provide you great benefits such as increased energy lose weight and get rid of certain illnesses like cold and flu.

Click here to start detox-Cleansing Now

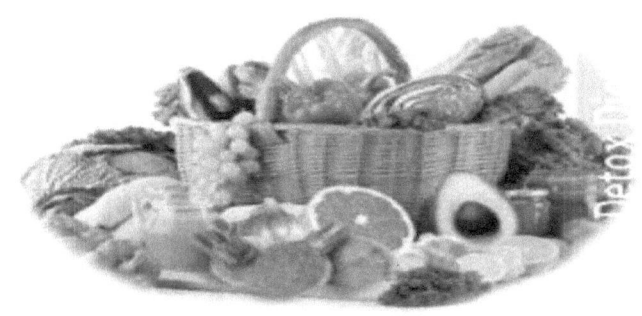

Detox Cleanse Weight Loss

They are ingredients that need to be incorporated into your Detox diet plan for you to detoxify your body and shed excess pounds.

There are 5 Amazing ingredients for detox and weight reduction:

1. Lemon: It helps cleanse the lymphatic system.

Among different essential phytonutrients it includes phosphorous that ensures the proper functioning of the anxious gadget and sodium that allows the toxins removal process and helps liver and gall bladder. Liver performs an essential role inside the fat metabolism.

Keeping your liver healthy will help you maintain your perfect weight.

Drink 1 glass of hot water with a thin slice of natural

lemon first thing in the morning to stimulate the liver.

2. Avocado: it is an essential source of glutathione, an anti-oxidant that protects liver. It binds with fats soluble toxins and makes them water-soluble so that they easily excreted from the body. For instance, it binds with alcohol and allows liver to effortlessly excrete it from the body hence protect liver from damage.

3. **Ginger**: It has a potential to stimulate the digestive device.

4. **Apple**: it is a source of vitamin C and quercetin that assist decrease the fats level in the body. It is also a good source of nutrition E, biotin, folic acid and other important phytonutrients and promotes healthy muscle tissues, nerves and respiratory system.

Pectin is a fiber found in apples as well as beets and citrus fruits. It binds to poisonous heavy metals, preservatives and additives and enables their excretion. These kinds of substances are a large burden for digestive machine and promote weight benefit.

5. Beetroot:

This is an extensively used detoxification resource.

It contains magnesium, manganese and folate. Beetroot is some of the excellent vegetable liver-cleansers. It additionally includes methionine that helps reduce cholesterol level.

[Click here to start detox-Cleansing Now](#)

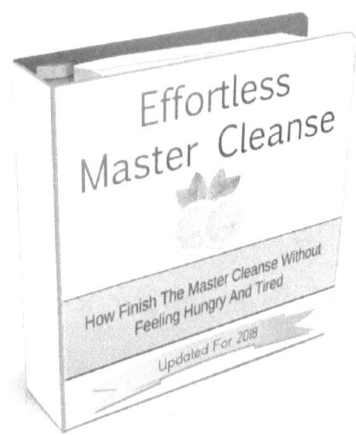

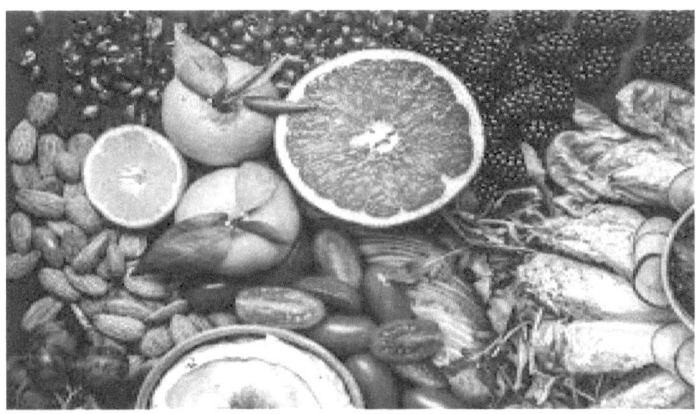

Want to Detox and shed pounds?

Get rid of these 3 ingredients for quicker weight loss

On the subject of successfully detoxifying and losing weight, you need to understand the dangers of these 3 ingredients: sugar, artificial sweeteners and processed foods. In other words, these ingredients may be responsible for your weight loss struggles. When you get rid of these 3 ingredients in your weight-reduction plan; you will quickly remove the accumulation of fat and pollutants--and shed more pounds quicker.

Sugar

Did you realize that an average Human being consumes half a pound of sugar daily! Simply because sugar is in almost everything they consumed, which means you can ingest lots of sugar without even knowing it.

I am certain you understand the damage sugar can do to your body system. Sugar contains nothing but empty energy. When you eat massive quantities of sugar (or meals that incorporate sugar), it reserved and stored in your body as fat.

Too much sugar in your weight loss plan makes you look and feel worn-out and fatigued-- and makes you gain excess weight. Sugar can also depress your metabolism and cause you to have diabetes. So it's important to lessen the "sugar highs." this is only possible if a great detox routine comes in.

With the aid of detoxifying your body system, you could reduce the sugar in your body quicker, do away with the build-up of fat and begin to lose weight.

Artificial "Low Calorie" Sweeteners

However before you run and purchase the ounces zero-calorie food regimen liquids, you must know this: synthetic sweeteners used in the ounces diet drinks and occasional-calorie drinks are poisonous chemicals. They're naturally produced. It is important for you to detoxify your body; you must stay away from artificial sweeteners as quickly as possible.

And in case, you're trying to lose weight faster through the use of synthetic/artificial sweeteners, think twice because synthetic sweeteners actually stimulates your appetite and make you consume more meals.

It's been proven that chemical sweeteners certainly raised immoderate urge for food and cravings for extra meals, as well as troubles your metabolism and hormones.

Truthfully, continual ailments and situations (including depression, tension, migraines, temper modifications and slow metabolism) are associated with how those artificial sweeteners interact with your body system.

These artificial sweeteners can virtually slow down the digestive, metabolic and hormonal imbalance, all of these may leads to excess weight gains.

Processed Meals

As you already know, processed ingredients are normally cheap, convenient and smooth to prepare. However unluckily, these ingredients are very bad for you. Food manufacturers are not going to give you a rundown of the bad substances they use to prepare the processed foods, so I will do it for you.

First many processed foods contain big amounts of Trans-fat. Trans-fat makes it difficult to lose weight and contributes to weight gains.

Trans - fat is one aspect you need to get away from as speedy as possible.

Secondly, a number of your preferred processed ingredients are loaded with excessive fructose corn syrup.

Excessive fructose corn syrup has been gaining attention recently due to the fact that it's far believed to be a main player within the rising epidemic of obesity.

Nutrition experts agree that excessive fructose corn syrup can be partly responsible for inflicting troubles along with your metabolism, which increases the likelihood of gaining weight. Cut down on processed foods and you will surely increase the chance of shedding weight.

Thirdly, manufacturers use chemical compounds in processed meals. These poisonous chemical substances contribute to gradual digestion and metabolic imbalances that make it difficult to lose weight.

I'm sure you can see the importance of Detox to cleanse these chemicals out of your body as **speedy as**

possible.

As you may see, the principle culprits of weight gain are these 3 foods: sugar, artificial sweeteners and processed foods.

You will shed pounds faster when you detox those dangerous substances out of your body System.

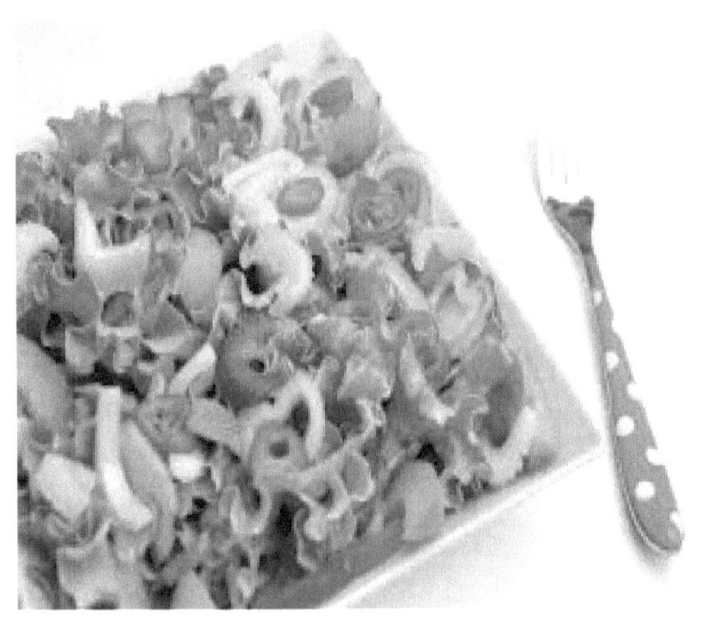

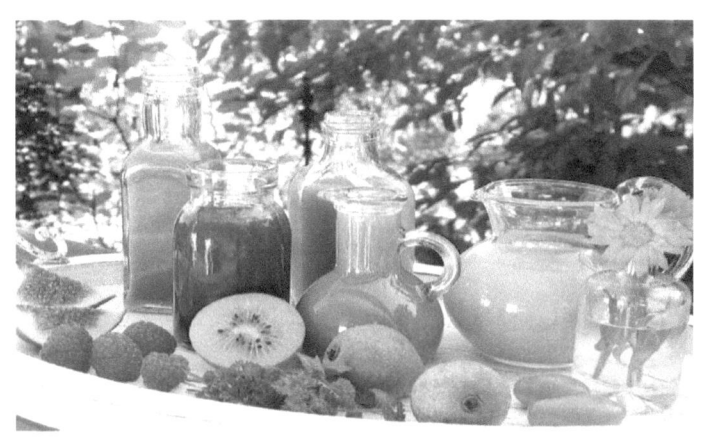

Smoothies Recipes For Detox and Protein weight loss plan

In case you hate counting calories or Weight Watcher points to bring your weight beneath control, or in case you are counting away so that you can lose a few pounds, that is right, simply stop.

Each article you ever read talks about the importance of eating 3-5 smaller food as the key to maintaining your weight beneath control.

But finding healthy food which might be satisfying and yummy each day may be an adventure.

However you can win the war of the burden with the assistance of a wide-kind of smoothie meals which offer nutrients, minerals, and antioxidants which might be flavourful and enjoyable.

Daily, health-conscious humans are adding smoothies to their diets.
Smoothies can be used any time of the day; breakfast, lunch, mid-meal snacks, or dinner.

Smoothies will help you integrate fruits and veggies in a wide variety of tasty and flavourful mixtures at the same time it will satisfy you with adequate vitamins and mineral you want for a meal plan that works great for your body.

Irrespective of your food regimen; be it a detox healthy eating plan, protein healthy eating plan, high, or low carb weight loss plan, smoothies can be seamlessly incorporated into your food regimen. Sincerely blend the substances wished o help you manipulate your eating regimen and hold your weight below control.

You may find out that smoothies will provide you with the basis of a weight loss program you may keep on with because they are both delicious and filling. And you can attempt a new smoothie every day.

Don't worry if you can't consider what to use, or how to begin. You are good to go with the Smoothie recipes listed below to proceed on your weight loss journey.

For People counting calories, start one, or both of these tomorrow: one for breakfast and one for a great afternoon snack

Apple Strawberry-Kiwi Smoothie

integrate in your blender

1 banana reduce in chunks.

1 kiwi peeled and reduce in 4 sections

1 cup of strawberries (if fresh approximately 4-6) you could additionally use frozen

1 cup of bloodless apple juice

1 Tbsp honey

combine the ingredients in your blender until smooth. If you use clean strawberries over frozen you may want to feature a touch extra apple juices to reach the consistency you want pleasantly. All your family members will love it. You may add a tsp of the chia seed Mila too, as a way to come up with even more brought vitamins and minerals.

Apple Carrot Smoothie

Perfect for lunch or as an afternoon snack, this recipe is likewise a low calorie smoothie, best to preserve your weight underneath manipulate.

Before you can make this
smoothie, take a bag of
carrots cut the tops and
scrub the pores and skin. You
do not need to peel the
carrots. Boil about 1-2 cups
of water, relying at the wide
variety of carrots getting
used and gently prepare
dinner till the carrots are
gentle.
Positioned the cooked carrots
in the fridge to kick back.

When it is time for lunch,
put it into your blender mix

2 cooked carrots (chilled)

1 cup of cold apple juice

1 tbsp Chia seed (awesome
supply of additional protein
consisting of coronary heart
healthful omega-three fatty
acids)

Click here to start detox-Cleansing Now

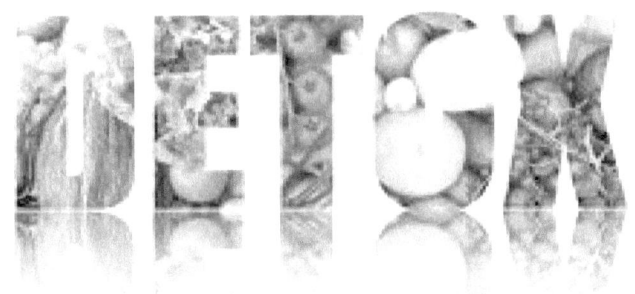

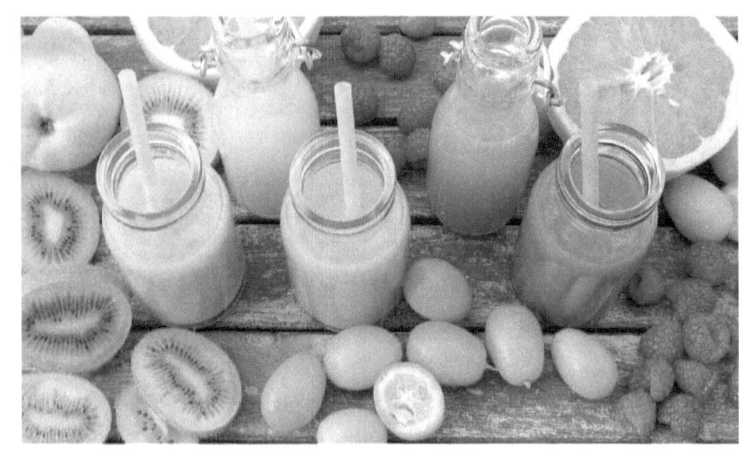

Detox food regimen: Juice Fasting Recipes

Juice fasting is gaining recognition as an amazing way to detoxify.

Many people are inquisitive about getting toxins out of

their body so as to live a
healthier life.

While toxins accumulate
inside the body, they
experience weakness and also
have a terrible immune
system.

Juice fasting, as a cleansing
technique, can assist people
to acquire better health and
greater power. It's far quite
simple to do as end result is
of great importance and all
that is required is a juicer.

For a newbie to embark on
juice fasting, it's far
essential to start off slowly

and to later increase the tempo at some point. By juice fasting, you're restricting your consumption to juices handiest. Fruit juice is high in sugar, so if you are a diabetic or in any other case in need of monitoring your sugar intake you have to be cautious of attempting a juice rapid with fruit juices.

To proceed on juice fasting you need to consult your health practitioner first.

Mores, do not do juice fasting for extended durations like more than three days, except your physician consents that it's safe for you to do so. Subsequently you can do pattern recipes which could help come up with concept of Juice combos and greens to use collectively:

Recipe 1: Vegetable Juice blend

2 Swiss chard leaves

1/2 beetroot

2 or 3 sprigs of watercress

3 carrots

1 celery stalk

Preparation:

Wash all with filtered or distilled water cut and put in juicer.

Recipe 2: Carrot-Apple Juice

2-3 inexperienced Apples

1 carrot

Sparkling basil leaves

Wash with filtered or distilled water cut and put in juicer.

Recipe three: Carrot Vegetable Juice

A handful of dandelion leaves

1 kale leaf

4 carrots

Clean mint, basil or coriander leaves

Wash with filtered or distilled water cut and put in juicer.

Recipe four: Peach Juice

2 or 3 peaches

Wash with filtered or distilled water cut and installed in juicer.

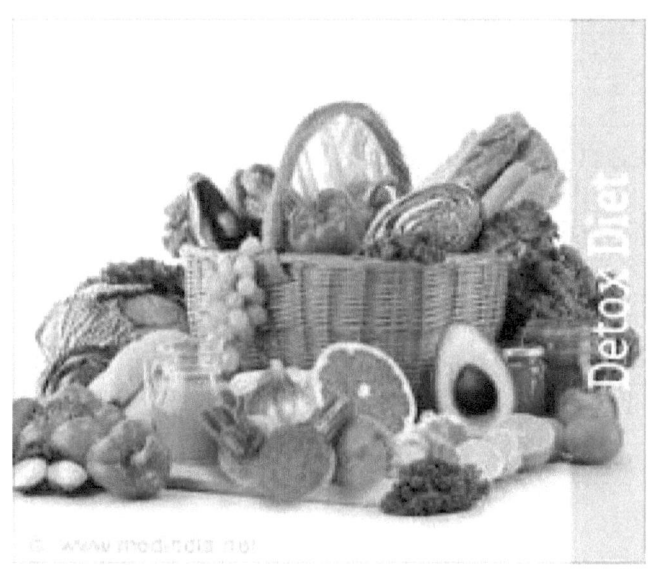

There are numerous exclusive kinds of juice fasts. A few diets name for fruit juices at the same time as others used much less sugary vegetable juices. You could come up with your own specific mixture of fruit and vegetable juice food plan recipes.

Five advantages of drinking Detox Tea.

Detox tea can be a very useful option to cleanse your body system. Detoxing has the capability to your health advantage together with clearing the pores and skin, soothing strain, and helping with weight reduction. Without an occasional detox, the body system can result in troubles associated with hormonal imbalances, kidney and liver problems, or brain disorder.

Let's test some of the fantastic **advantages of detox tea:**

Eliminate all body pollution

The body's cells and tissues will see an herbal construct-up of chemical compounds, environmental pollution, insecticides and heavy metals over the years. This may have a negative effect at the body as it lowers the capacity to fight disease. A regular detox can help to enhance the immune device and cleanse the liver obviously.

The more effective liver facilitates to lower sickness-inflicting inflammation.

Increase strength and mental alertness

A normal drink of detox tea can assist to reinforce electricity that is useful for eliminating the feeling of brain fog, temper swings and fatigue. Additionally, certain teas like mint and rosemary can be beneficial for enhancing all-spherical mental alertness.

Weight loss

The fine gain of boosting power tiers and metabolism can imply you are left feeling that rather more energized. Any profitable detox tea will encompass energetic substances like nutrients and minerals, HCA (hydroxycitric acid), catechins and flavonoids. HCA is specifically helpful because it has the capability to suppress the appetite to further help in the manner of weight reduction.

additionally, the herbal and healthful substances is that this sort of tea are a lot extra powerful at retaining the stomach complete in comparison to ingesting dangerous snacks.

Enhance digestion

Detox tea is remarkable for improving digestion and mainly beneficial for troubles like constipation, nausea, bloating and fuel. The Detox technique will assist your body to take away the build-up of waste substances stored inside the belly.

True skin

Just like having a poor impact at the body's cells and problems, the build-up of pollutants will even attack the skin. Truly being out and about can lead to the pores and skin absorbing pollutants that leave the skin dull and dry. A detox tea in the morning can be a beneficial option to nourish the body and assist to combat-everyday body pollution.

Detox tea is a simple solution to cleanse the system. It's very easy to prepare at domestic and maximum teas taste splendid. Additionally, the benefits are even more effective when mixed with a wholesome weight loss plan and habitual workout.

Click here to try Red Tea Detox for better result Now

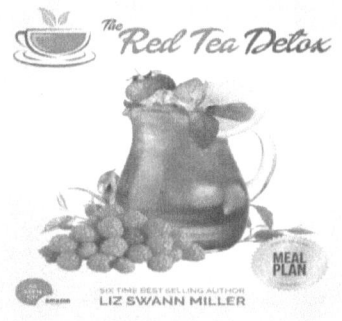

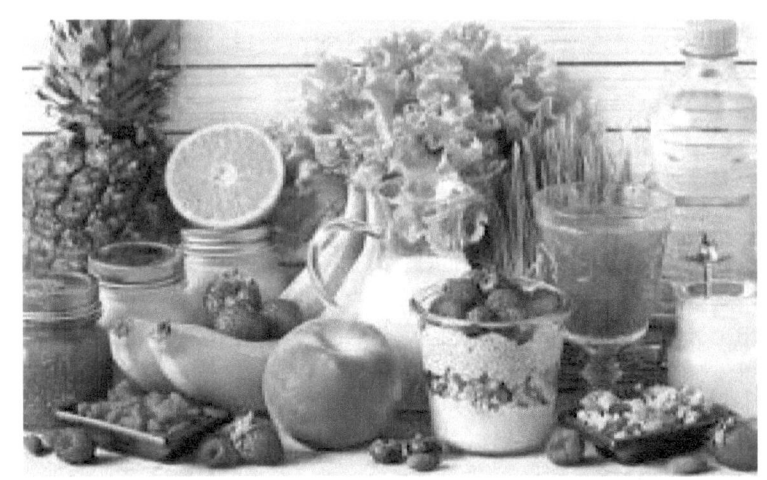

10 Powerful Steps to Safe Detoxification

We live in a grand time of technological development. Computers, the net, cellular telephones, virtual cameras and DVDs. but the human body has not 'beefed up' with technology. Humans really shouldn't eat Technology!

However that is occurring nowadays as a result of the onslaught of chemical compounds in our meals and environments, and with the impending threat of chemical struggle. Secondly, your physical body is mysteriously functioning internally exactly the manner human bodies functioned 10,000 years in the past; due to the fact that our bodies these days are the same as in the past, it's miles vital to consume, drink, and live similar to in years beyond - centuries beyond. But cutting-edge societies are adopting one of the most unnatural lives recognised to mankind. Most cancers costs and cardiovascular sickness within the U.S. on my own are the various highest inside the international as a result of technology interfering with our meals supply and residing environments.

SO WHY DETOX?

Have you ever washed greasy dishes without hot water or dish soap? The dishes don't get clean, do they? While poisonous metals and chemical food components get inside your body, it takes a strong "purifier" to scrub your body smooth from the inside out. The mixture of nutrients and minerals through detoxification paintings on this style to dispose of toxins out of your body tissues and frame organs, out of fats deposits, and within your bloodstream.

Herbal cleansing is important to do away with your body toxins, and protects it from re-depositing them someplace else within the body system.

Pollution inclusive of lead, mercury, and the facet outcomes of aspartame's through-products of formic acid and formaldehyde, block vitamins from stepping into everyday body cells inside the identical style a lead protect blocks radiation in the course of an x-ray.

If toxins are present inside your frame, oxygen and the body's "meals supply" cannot get inner your cells to deliver wished vitamins, nor can the cells' waste merchandise get out. Sicknesses, which include cancer, now have an environment wherein to shape. Whilst these toxins are removed, your body structure can then be repair and gained healthy stability.

Detect, get rid of, AND repair

The fundamental philosophy behind any effective detox application is to identify, remove, and repair.
You've got to become aware of what pollution are at the

foundation of your health troubles.

Discover = hair analysis
Put off the toxins with the aid of cleansing your body system.
Do away with Toxins = detoxification

Restore misplaced nutrients.

Repair = dietary supplements

Like pealing the layers off an onion, as every layer is removed through detoxing, the underlying layers screen what is simply behind sickness symptoms.

The deeper you move in the direction of disposing of the 'centre' of the hassle, recuperation will become long-time period truth.

Click here to start detox-cleansing now

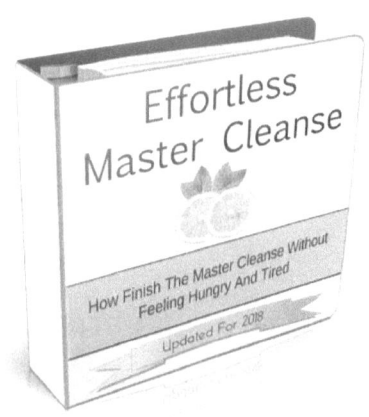

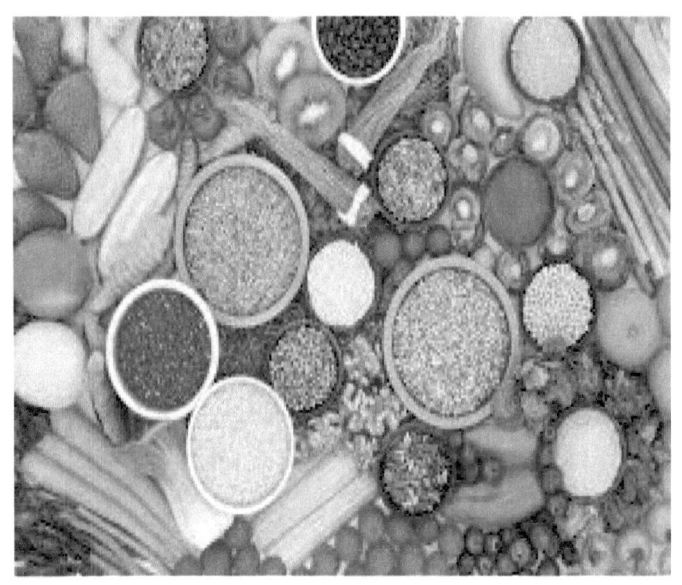

TEN STEPS TO DETOXING

Begin with cleansing your body of all residual chemical toxins and see if any unfavourable fitness signs continue to be. Try these steps for yourself, and inside 30 days your symptoms need to enhance if not absolutely disappear.

The ten Steps:

- Do away with all chemical compounds from your diet.
- Learn how to 'examine' your body System.
- Start recording any fitness adjustments.
- Get a hair evaluation.
- Be satisfied with yourself.
- Detoxify restore depleted nutrients.
- Exercise to get your body relaxed.

- Consume 75% uncooked ingredients at each meal.
- Drink water, water, water.
- Manage your lifestyles.

Do not neglect the reality that healing from ailment and contamination takes faith, personal power, and perseverance. Curing infection and degenerative sicknesses with a thoughts-body approach might be taken into consideration and useless whilst in comparison to modern high tech prescriptions, however it is essential that human beings take into account that the roots of ailment and their remedies are as the body itself, and recovery begins with SELF.

Detoxification is the total Prevention of all Health Issues

Detoxifying the body structure has come to be an apparent key preventive degree to all styles of health issues. On account that maximum folks are busy, and not able or unwilling to hold a strict food plan in order to absolutely get rid of all of the pollutants from their body frame. We've got chemical compounds build up in our bodies every day. Seeing that those chemicals aren't harmful in small quantities, only in larger accumulated amounts, we don't note side results till we are a great deal older. A proper, even if is occasional, detox weight-reduction plan is necessary to relieve our bodies of harmful pollution and chemical substances, and hold a healthy, everyday, and long-lived lifestyles.

The primary concept of a detox food plan is to get rid of almost all unwanted substances out of your body system and restrict the body to simplest water and vegetables for a few days; typically around five or 6 days is adequate.

Maximum detox diets then permit for a gradual re-introduction of different ingredients, step by step. Detox Diets usually restrict foods from your weight loss program which are said to have harmful pollution.

Together with this a detox food plan should then flush the present pollutants out of the body. Detox weight loss plan essentially offers the liver and different organs a threat to trap up and dispose of all of the toxins.

That is done through our sweat, feces, and urine.

Our bodies virtually can't deal with the ordinary daily ingestion of chemical substances.

Chemicals come from ingredients, as cited earlier but also have a huge sort of different resources. Although we do not realize what meals is the cause of all of it, we do realize that insecticides, heavy metals, together with mercury and lead, and the chemicals in cigarettes and the air we breathe, all inside our bodies via our lungs or belly and might result in an excessive building up. These chemicals in small quantities are innocent; it's the everyday ingestion and building up of them which could lead to degenerative sicknesses. One not unusual detox weight loss plan is the mixture of not anything however ends result and water for a given length. The merchandising of chemical substances being metabolized through our bodies may be helped with sure nutrients, herbs and supplements. A few supplements will assist the mobilization of pollutants in our fat and other toxin deposits located at some stage in the frame. Given that our bodies rid themselves of chemical compounds via sweat, sauna cures can also provide an extremely good benefit. There are numerous different diets and detox treatments, these are only a few not unusual methods. Regular body cleansing is a superb preventative motion and promotes a healthier present and destiny.

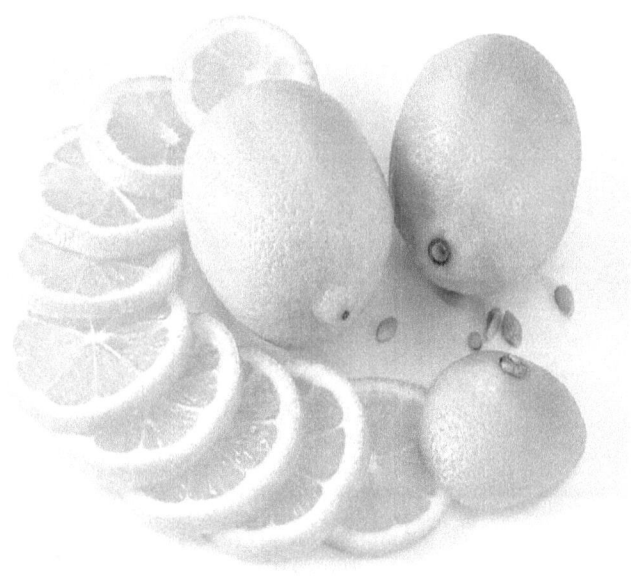

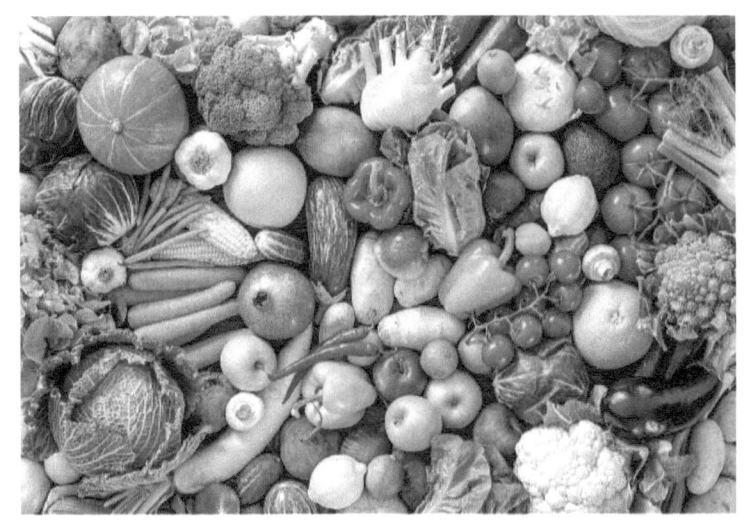

Herbal Detox Diets For long term health

With lot of chemical substances in the whole thing we eat, it's far pretty tough to hold all of the junk out of our systems and most effective consume the healthy stuff. The coolest news is that even after consuming dangerous meals, even though many pollution stay in our bodies for some time, it is constantly possible to do away with them. For clearer pores and skin, extended power, and higher health common detoxing diets are becoming increasingly more famous. The concept is that these diets flush the machine especially, the liver, kidneys and colon of pollution that are acquired through a normal food regimen. Maximum detox diets typically eliminate toxins from our body anywhere from one week to a month. However to extend those diets can offer a few awesome life-style recommendation to everybody, even those no longer committing to a complete detox weight loss plan. Considering the wide variety of chemical substances in fast meals, junk food, or even food and drinks which could seem healthy, like milk for instance, toxins need to be methodically flushed out of the body so often.

The easy however handiest way to detoxify is by using drinking plenty of water. Water flushes and purifies the body of any junk inside it. An amazing manner to test for proper hydration is by paying attention to the colour of your urine. Clean urine signifies right hydration however extra yellow urine signifies that you have to drink plenty/excess water. A terrific manner to ensure right hydration is via spotting a water bottle and consuming from it whenever you're thirsty in place of opting for bad liquids. Even liquids that seem herbal, like apple juice, may additionally have preservatives and artificial sugars so sticking to water all through detox is the pleasant guess. Drinking tea, especially inexperienced tea additionally has many advantages for detoxification.

Next, there is the consumption of end result, veggies, and herbal grains.

These vitamins are without problems processed by way of the body and maximum detox diets include excessive intake of those gadgets. Red meats, dairy, and greasy foods have to be averted throughout the detox duration. For protein during the eating regimen, fish, fowl and nuts can be fed on. Green vegetables, lentils, and brown rice are also splendid alternatives. Exceptionally smoking, drugs, and the consumption of alcohol ought to be averted for the duration of detoxification due to the fact this stuff need to be taken into consideration pollutants.

Although the food plan itself is important, exercising is also a totally critical part of a detoxification process. Whilst exercise, the body sweats out sure toxins that won't in any other case expel. The accelerated body temperature throughout exercising also allows purify the body frame.

Exercise 3 times per week for at the least half of an hour on every occasion is sufficient to purify the body but extra exercise is usually accurate. The workout itself doesn't want to be strenuous; whatever that will increase coronary heart beat and body temperature will do the activity.

There are numerous better-finances alternatives for detoxing as well, inclusive of detox beverages and "internal body organ cleansers" but the recommendations above work simply as properly, if not higher.

The idea of the weight loss plan is really to eliminate extra toxins out while flushing the body of something dangerous that already exists internally.

If detox diets are accomplished often, the dieter will find himself or herself with elevated power, long time health benefits, and clearer skin.

Click here to start detox-cleansing now

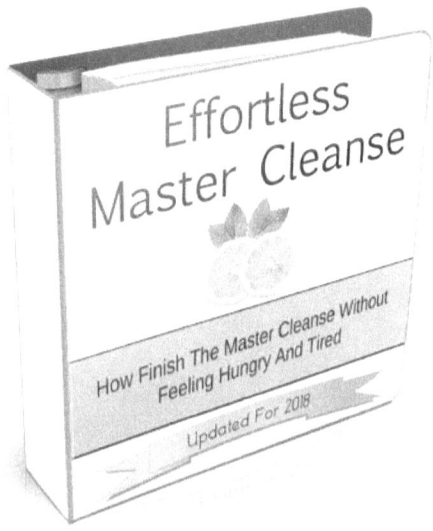

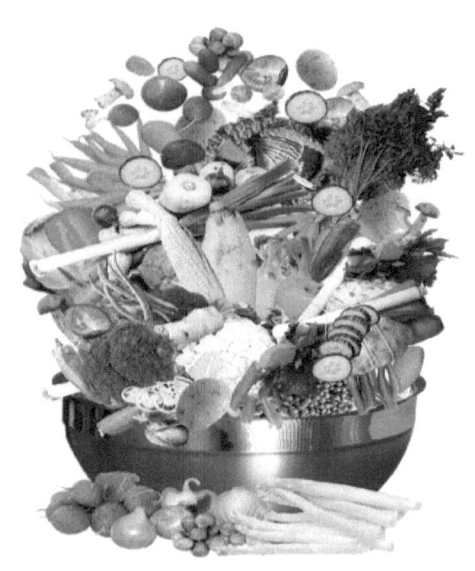

7 home made Detox drinks for weight reduction

These Self made Detox drinks for weight loss are a natural way to melt the fat rapidly.

Detoxification gets rid of toxins and facilitates you to

reach your weight loss dreams in a short period of time. So certainly it's a good idea to detox your body on a solid foundation.

It's important to note that ingesting best detoxification beverages into your body for number of days will make you to accelerate your ordinary weight loss to a detox weight loss plan.

Please seek an advice from your doctor before you start any type of lengthy-term or drastic detox cleanse plan.

With that being said here are **7 homemade detox drinks that will help you lose weight:**

Tea: Tea is a natural detox drink that expels pollutants out of your body system. Dandelion tea, inexperienced tea, peppermint tea, and ginger tea are especially effective in supporting weight loss. Drink three-five cups of tea each day to assist your weight loss efforts.

Cranberry Juice: Cranberry

juice enhances the body's metabolism that is crucial to converting fat into power as opposed to extra weight. In conjunction with ingesting Q wawa fruits and vegetables, ingesting cranberry juice is a totally powerful manner to lose weight. In addition this detox drink also allows cleanse nicotine and alcohol out of your body within four days. Drink at least 32 oz of a 100% natural organic cranberry juice every day.

Cabbage Juice: Cabbage may be very effective for

detoxifying your liver. And because your liver is accountable for the detoxification of your entire body, its form a crucial part of your detox and diet plan. If you have a juicer, juice up a few cabbage, carrots and pears for a deliciously clean detox drink.

Cabbage Broth: For a satisfying warm drink, simmer a head of cabbage together with carrots, onions and a pinch of salt, then strain and drink. You may additionally include different greens to p.c. greater vitamins into this hot detox drink, which is very effective for detoxifying your liver.

Cucumber and Lemon: This might appear like a stunning aggregate, but the results of these components was examined via expert nutritionists and concluded to be a powerful detox and weight loss drink. All you have to do is use a blender to mix 1 cucumber sliced into tiny portions and half lemon juice. Drink at least 2 times daily. This detox drink boosts your metabolism, which is important for losing weight speedily, and you will notice the way it fill you with energy.

Master Cleanse Lemonade: This is probably the most famous detox drink for weight loss in the industry. It was made famous by way of celebrities like Angelina Jolie and Beyoncé Knowles due to the fact it's far an exceptionally effective detox drink for weight reduction and for improving your pores and skin complexion. This is an ideal self-made detox drink to lose weight rapidly.

Mix lemon juice
Organic maple syrup and a dash of cayenne pepper into a glass of water.
Sip in this drink all day for satisfactory outcomes.
Salt Water Cleanse: at the beginning of your detox, you would possibly need to do a salt water detox to cleanse your digestive system and prepare your body for weight loss. do that on a day when you have lots of time to stay

domestic near the toilet as it will run via your body very quickly. Blend 1 to 2 tablespoons of natural sea salt into one quarter of lukewarm water. Do not use table salt; it will not give the best results.

Stir or shake till the salt is dissolved.

Drink and then relax. Most people feel a bowel movement inside between 30 minutes to two hours and several more as observe. Once you've got your body cleansed and repair it by consuming yogurt to top off the useful micro organism on your digestive tract, drink juice, and consume clean, soft-cooked, steamed veggies.

In addition to these detox diet make sure to consume lots of greens, culmination and entire grain foods that fill you up and give you the great chance for speedy losing weight.

Click here to start detox-cleansing now

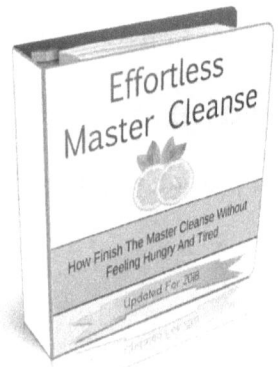

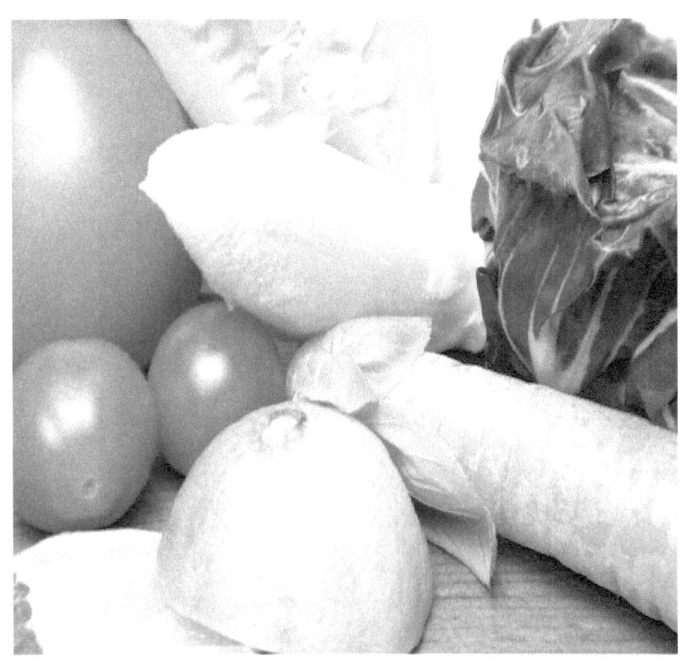

Healthy weight reduction: The Detox food plan manner

Permanent weight loss Equals wholesome weight reduction

Permanent   and   wholesome

weight   reduction   can't

simplest   improve   ones.

However it could additionally be an imperative part of growing common bodily, mental, emotional and non secular properly-being. But, many weight reduction techniques train the victim (You!) to do all the incorrect things, and eat all the incorrect ingredients, main to rebound weight gain. In case you lose weight in a healthful manner, then you definitely weight loss could be everlasting.

Weight Watchers Damages Metabolism

I've visible so many people going to a program like Weight Watchers absolutely break their metabolism by means of losing greater muscle than fat. They get applauded every week after they enhance their weight reduction via dropping muscle. Ultimately, this character ends up gaining the load returned because of the metabolic gradual-down because of the lack of muscle that is discouraging to mention the least.

Food regimen and Detox weight loss

No wholesome detox weight loss plan is complete without a nicely-balanced weight-reduction plan of real meals! I propose a colourful Mediterranean weight loss plan this has changed to be low glycemic index. Organising a wholesome weight-reduction plan does not suggest eliminating all carbs; nor does it suggest stocking your shelf with low-fat diet meals. As a substitute, you should intake a weight loss plan full of lean proteins, lots of non-starchy veggies, and constrained quantities of beans, healthful fruits and nuts. Non-obligatory could a few limited amounts of entire grains. Of course, no detox food regimen could be complete without masses of natural water.

Movement and Detox weight reduction

Further to a nutritious weight loss program and lots of water, motion is also crucial for detox weight reduction. Irrespective of what sort of motion you experience, the essential component is to get going! Strive strolling five times every week for about half-hour. No longer only are you getting exercising and burning energy, however you also are shifting lymph, and stimulating blood glide via your tissues - crucial for correct detoxing.

In case you resides in a northern weather wherein walking out of doors might be dangerous within the iciness because of slippery conditions, most department stores welcome exercising walkers. If taking walks is not your element, take into account turning into a member of the nearby health club. There are normally many aerobic alternatives which include motorcycles, elliptical machines, stair stepping machines, treadmills, etc. in addition, most gyms offer weight machines, loose weights, balls, and many others. Maximum gyms additionally provide lessons which include spin training, aerobics lessons, and extra.

When you have to choose among aerobic and resistance, the technological know-how suggests that you will burn extra fat within the end with resistance workout, specifically in case you do big compound actions that work massive muscle mass in corporations, spiking your coronary heart price. This high-intensity approach will increase your metabolism for over 48 hours. So doing each resistance and cardio exercise is great, but relaxation assured that an easy one hundred fifty minute per week on foot software in conjunction with a scientifically-based detox weight-reduction plan diet regime will paintings

if you simply cannot seem to go it by myself, an

investment in a non-public teacher can be really worth your even as you try to obtain a few healthful fat burning. Even though non-public trainers may additionally appear costly, they are able to often save you injuries by ensuring you use the proper shape.

I recognize that harm may be a far-off idea for you proper now, but believe me, an damage can truly set again your weight loss and belly fat lowering goals dramatically. Consider no longer being capable of exercise in any respect! In preference to exerting maximal attempt, the higher choice is to dial it lower back a bit to prevent harm. Educate don't pressure is the watchword.

I really like my private trainers to have a "contact of gray" if you understand what I mean. This increases the probability that they've treated their very own schooling injuries. Personal enjoy with injuries makes for a wiser private trainer who can higher at assist you keep away from harm that could stop your weight reduction progress.

Weight loss program drugs Are Crap

You understand from reading my food plan drugs article than ninety nine.99% of the weight-reduction plan capsules available are natural crap! The simplest weight-reduction plan tablets that without a doubt paintings without a rebound effect are ones that nourish the detoxing pathways of the frame, so the liver receives decongested and fats is burned faster. you may see lots of other blessings too, digestion enhancing, pores and skin and eyes getting clearer, rashes and pores and skin conditions spontaneously clearing up, and aches and pains going away. The high-quality side effect of which includes detox nutrition in your fats-burning plan is this: whilst you are toxic, your frame keeps a number of water. When you Detox diet you lose that extra water weight quickly, without dehydrating yourself, accelerating your slimming and weight reduction. In this situation, the water loss is healthful, as it isn't from the use of diuretic diets tablets, but happening clearly from having more healthy, much less-poisonous cells.

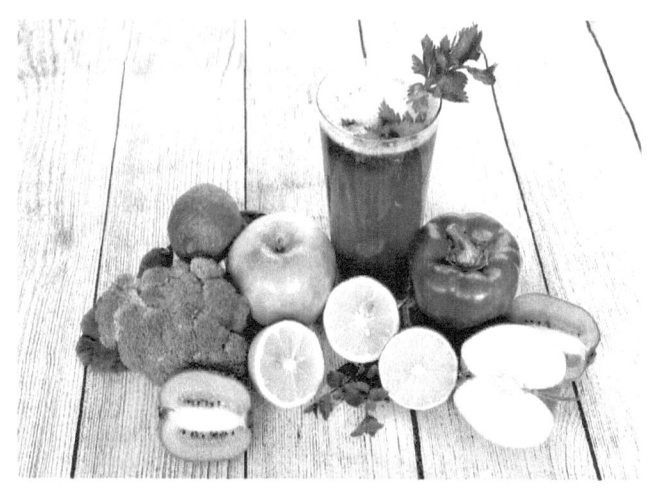

Fad Detox Diets increase Toxicity and Impair fats burning

Fasting on only fruit, the "master Cleanse", the "Popcorn diet" and other unhealthy fad detox diets virtually all fall down for 2 reasons:

First, your body needs an extensive range of vitamins in order to detoxify and excrete pollutants. When you are on a remarkable constrained mono food regimen or fad just like the grasp Cleanse, you honestly impair the cleansing procedure, impeding your fat burning!

Secondly, toxins and their toxic metabolites flow into the body and get redeposit inside the tissues inflicting toxicity complications and flu-like signs. Unknowing clients of the fashion detox diets frequently expect that their headaches, body-aches, and runny noses are sign that their fad eating regimen is running; however in reality this indicates that they are lacking important nutritional substances for proper detox.

I can't emphasize sufficient how dangerous these fad diets are. They usually cause impair fats-burning and detoxing also increase toxicity.

A wholesome Detox eating regimen method

Though there are many weight loss techniques out there, but for first-rate consequences we suggest a healthy detoxing weight-reduction plan technique that includes movement, an ingesting gadget for existence, and plenty of tissue cleansing dietary guide for quick results. A detox diet for life approach a non-fad detox food regimen that elements you with the protein, fiber, and different nutrients to nourish wholesome body systems and metabolic detoxification pathways so your body can detox each day, for the relaxation of your system.

When your aim is detox weight loss, then observe those identical standards with decreased caloric consumption, and recall supplementing your healthy entire-food detox diet with a scientifically-based supplement that nourishes the metabolic detox pathways for better results.

<u>Click here to start detox-cleansing now</u>

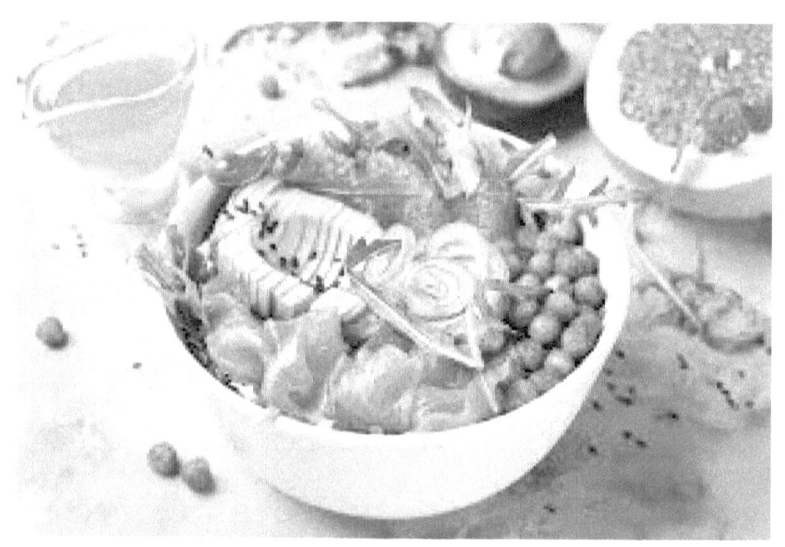

Recipes for a Detox weight loss program and Your Oxidation charge

Knowing your oxidation rate is a vital piece of facts for your fitness. Your oxidation rate in simple phrases is how rapid do you burn meals? A few humans burn food slowly while others burn food speedily. In either case knowing this essential piece of information, has a huge impact on matching you with the best diet recipes for your body detox and your health.

A person who burns food rapid is known as a fast oxidizer and a person who burns food slowly is referred to as a slow oxidizer.

A fast oxidizer needs more gradual burning food including a weight-reduction plan with more high fine exact fats and oil. The sluggish burning meals are great in shape for the fast oxidizer as that individual will maintain strength.

In contrast the slow oxidizer may have a weight loss program of extra rapid burning food along with grain merchandise, however less of the high fine fats and oil. So there may be a large distinction between the two in phrases in their metabolic wishes.

In case your eating regimen is not matching your

oxidation rate you no longer getting the proper matching food for the velocity at which your system burns food. This matching element for correct diet is one of the main keys to desirable health.

Now that you realize your oxidation charge is important, how do you discover your oxidization charge?
The secret is your hair; despite the fact that your hair is lifeless it is a storage website for all your

macro minerals, hint minerals and toxic metals. As the hair grows out these minerals and pollution are deposited in the hair over a three to 4 month period. Through a hair mineral check and with the expertise of a laboratory that examines your hair nicely, you may determine your oxidation rate. As soon as this vital piece of information is understood, you could pin point your actual weight loss program for you and handiest you.

No more guess work! And for the folks that had the intuition that all ingredients do not affect everybody identically, bravo you have been right and the two oxidation costs are why. An example might be if you're a fast oxidizer than masses of grains, and end result are not a fantastic preference due to grains and end result burn in no time and for immediate oxidation sustained energy can't be possible. The fast oxidizer will continually be hungry now not lengthy when they devour. I recognise there are those pronouncing it really is me, I get hungry an hour after I devour and the reason is an incorrect eating regimen.

Now in assessment if the short oxidizer eats sluggish burning food like eggs, olive oil, butter or some nuts (as an example) than sustained energy will manifest and the want to eat will slow down. Sluggish oxidizers have the reverse impact; they need and can consume faster burning meals which will preserve their power ranges.

In an effort to simplify this, there are a few people who are like an automobile speeding along on a toll road that burns gasoline very speedy. (Fast oxidizer) And the alternative is the automobile that is using slowly down a side road. (Slow oxidizers)

If we take the analogy one step in addition it's like a car that needs unleaded gasoline but you're putting in some diesel gasoline combined with some unleaded gasoline. It is the wrong fuel! It'll paintings but not at its first-class and over the years upkeep could be needed.

Now that the idea of your oxidation and weight loss plan has been explained let's talk about detox weight loss program. The excitement phrase "detox diet" is being thrown available often but until you already know your oxidation rate you will be ingesting the wrong meals or the incorrect food lots of the time. Detox diets must match a person's oxidation rate.

In this article I gift to you a sample meal plan for both gradual and speedy oxidizers.

Recipes for Detox diet:

Breakfast for gradual oxidizer:

2 eggs with spinach omelette, in 1 teaspoon of olive oil or butter

1 slice Ezekiel bread simple

1/four cup of blueberries

Breakfast for instant oxidizer:

2 eggs with spinach omelette, in 3 tablespoons of olive oil or butter

2 links organic turkey sausage

1 celery stalk with almond butter

In this example the slow oxidizer breakfast has less fats and oil of their meal and is permitted to have an excessive first-class grain product in addition to a small amount of fruit. The sluggish oxidizer will burn that meals slowly and sustain electricity via out the morning.

In contrast the quick oxidizer desires extra olive oil or butter in their food plan and greater fats and oil in the almond butter and turkey sausage. This mixture of meals will burn slowly for the quick oxidizer and preserve that character with sustained strength via out the morning.

Lunch for the slow oxidizer:

4 ounces Roasted chicken Breast, very mild butter and garlic
1 cup steamed carrots with 1 teaspoon of butter and sea salt
Half of cup brown rice

Lunch for the fast oxidizer:

4 oz. Roasted chook thighs, made with modest amount of butter and garlic
1 cup of steamed carrots with 3 tablespoons of butter and sea salt
Pecans 6-8

In this example again you may see that the gradual oxidizer has lots less fats and oil than the quick oxidizer.
Both have their protein and vegetable. Sluggish has the grain (brown rice) the fast has extra fats and oil.
(Darkish meat fowl, butter and pecan) The slow has the chook breast a whole lot less fat.

Dinner for the gradual oxidizer:

Four oz Flounder broiled with garlic and splash of lemon
Swiss chard with cranberries

Small quantity of olive oil
Sweet potato simple

Dinner for fast oxidizer:

4oz.Flounder with butter and garlic

Swiss chard with almonds and butter and olive oil

Candy potato with 3 tablespoons of butter

Once more we see that the sluggish oxidizer may have flounder with lemon and the gradual may have the cranberries and simple sweet potato. The fast has the flounder with butter which has extra fats and additionally the short has more butter at the candy potato and fat in the almonds.

Those recipes are examples of the distinction between the oxidation prices of sluggish and rapid individuals. Without knowing the speed your body burns food all the detox diets within the global can have very little high quality impact or even may be harmful.

For instance the popular lemon detox food regimen isn't an amazing desire for immediate oxidizers as their rate of oxidation requires slower burning food. Lemon is a fruit and it burns very fast and this kind of detox routine need to be avoided.

Matching your body with the precise detox food plan and the suitable dietary supplements and existence style adjustments are so much greater healthful for the long term than fad diets or fad liquid berry beverages.

Now not only will you detox efficaciously and competently your correct diet will have wonderful outcomes on weight reduction and weight benefit. It's quite simple, recognise your oxidation rate!

I would love to quick mention that the rule of thumb is to avoid foods which have artificial additives or that have low nutrients. The best foods are those ones in their natural form without any additives.

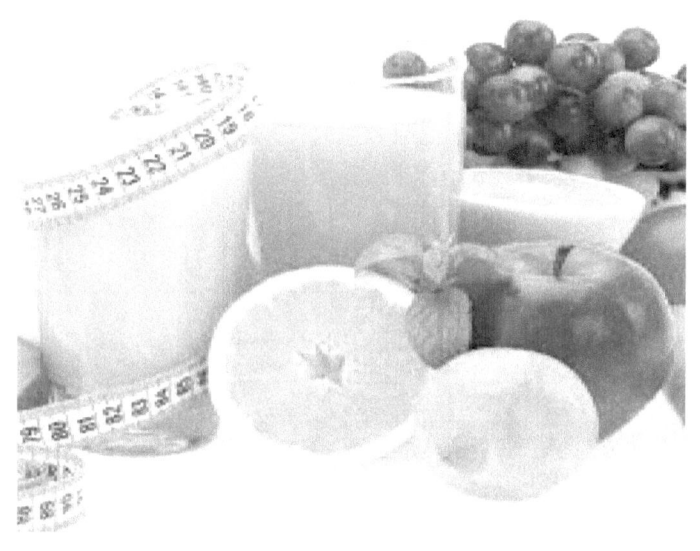

What's A HAIR analysis?

A hair analysis determines precisely what chemical substances are inside of you, which include radiation. Everyday scientific laboratory checks do not discover deep tissue toxins or nutrient depletions the same way a hair analysis does.

The protein in hair fibre holds the composition of the body tissues for a permanent period. Through studying your hair fibre composition, you may tell what toxins have gathered within the body tissues and what vitamins and minerals are depleted or too abundant causing imbalances in body function.

By means of detoxifying unnatural chemical compounds and through replacing particular vitamins according to individual needs; right fitness can be restored with the use of nutrients. The human hair analysis factors out those levels, making the hair analysis the exceptional device available.

Take the time to determine at which factor you may have gotten off beam nutritionally and what 'poisons' you have been exposed to.

Detox your body of all environmental and meals chemicals you might have ingested throughout your lifetime.

Restore depleted nutrients via proper supplements and complete ingredients.

Pollutants are at the foundation of most sicknesses, and once they're removed, your health will properly be restored.

A powerful detoxification plan eliminates the source of disorder signs and symptoms, along with aspartame or radiation poisoning, detoxifies poisonous residue from the frame, and replaces specific vitamins to regain a state of well being. Cleansing the body removes

toxins and unwanted chemicals
fast out of your blood
streams, body tissues and
support organs plus all fat
stored inside the
bloodstream, removal of those
pollutants through the bowels
and pores of the body.

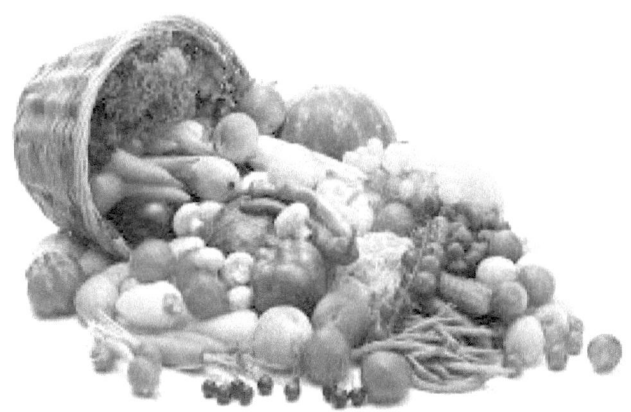

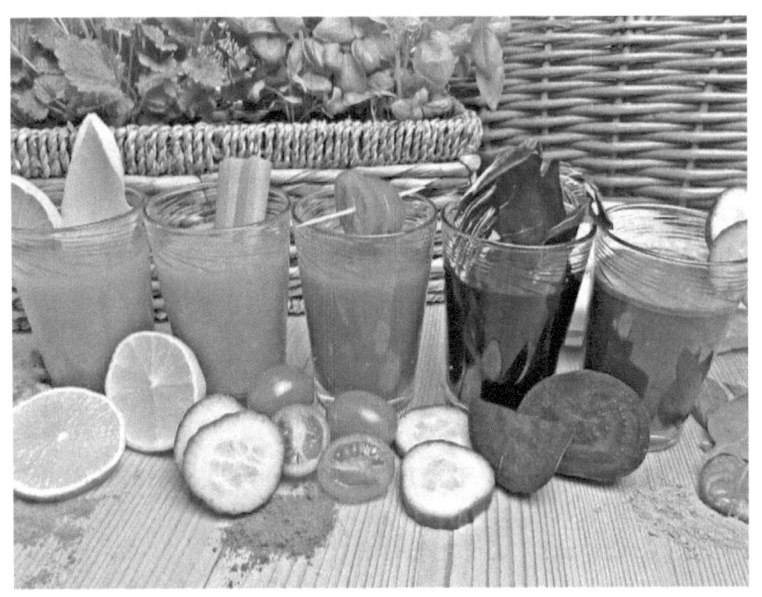

Detoxification and Your health - The bodies 7 Channels of elimination!

If you want to be healthy you need to recognize the seven systems that the body uses to eliminate waste and toxic matters. When those structures are working perfectly the end result is good health. When they are compromised all types of complications can result. For you to understand detoxification process you must have deep knowledge of body's channels of elimination.

When the body system confronts a toxin or overseas substance it uses those channels of removal to purge the toxin out of the body as quick as possible.

The key to great health is get hold of those 7 channels of elimination just like the back of your hand and doing everything viable to make them function properly.

In 1904 a Russian Naturopathic physician by way of the call of Eli Metchnikof located that the body system might recycle any toxin that no longer able to purging. Inside the recycling process the body could make use of all 7 channels of removal to try to get the poisonous substance eliminated out of the body.

That is essential to apprehend due to the fact that your health has been compromised so one or more of the bodies channels of elimination are not working effectively.

Majority of people can't even call the body's seven channels of elimination. If your health is important to you, do whatever you can to study and understand these seven vital cleansing systems.

The Bodies Seven Channels Of Elimination

<u>Liver</u> - The Liver is our body's factory that metabolizes meals, filters pollutants and converts substances into materials which are needed in all parts of the body system. The liver is certainly one of the largest and the most important organs of the body. When Liver is healthy it will save vitamins, sugars, fats and other vitamins from the food that you eat. The Liver builds chemical compounds that your body needs to stay

healthy and break down harmful substances, like alcohol and other toxic (poisonous) chemical compounds. It additionally gets rid of waste products out of your blood and makes sure that your body has the proper amount of other chemical substances that it desires.

Learn about the Liver via picking up a primary eBook on fitness and complement thus.

Lungs - The LUNGS are in control of breathing you need to take very good care of it.

The best way to take care of the lungs is through exercises.

You can keep your lung healthy if you don't smoke.

Smoking isn't appropriate for any part of your body, and your lungs specifically hate it. Deep breathing of sparkling air is the great exercising for the LUNGS. Kindly spend 15 mins every day doing deep breathing exercises for you to keep it healthy.

Lymphatic System - The

Lymphatic is the body's filter system which supports the role of immune system. Regular exercising is the high-quality treatment that your lymphatic system needs.

A healthy lymphatic system filters out bacteria's and other foreign micro organisms out of the body.

A natural herb by the name of arabanogalactan is an herbal cleanser of the lymphatic system.

Blood - The blood is a liquid organ which transfers and transports substances throughout the body. Its supplies the needed nutrition to all the areas that are in need.

Red Clover and Chlorella are brilliant natural cleansers of the blood system.

Habitual routine exercise stimulates the blood system and assists the body in getting rid of waste.

Skin - The skin is the largest body organ.

When you sweat naturally you assist in cleaning the skin, preserving it, make it more elastic and healthy. Going to a Sauna and sweating is a first best health routine for the pores and skin.

Colon - The colon is essential to effective health as it serves the function of transporting waste out of the body system. Proper hydration of the digestion system will enhance Colon health. This can be carried out daily by drinking plenty of clean water in your body weight.

Hydrating the colon through Colon Hydrotherapy is another means to re-establishing good health.

Kidneys - The kidneys produce urine which is the waste in the body.

Your probabilities of developing a kidney stone on your lifetime are 1 in 10? In 1995, greater than 3 million humans within the United State had a few kind of kidney circumstance which includes kidney contamination, kidney stones or mostly cancers. Extra than 300,000 humans beings had been afflicted by renal failure every year and go through dialysis or look ahead to a kidney transplant.

Often times kidney problems are the end result of dehydration. You must indulge in drinking plenty of clean water always to avoid kidney diseases.

A natural complement that cleanses and offers wanted nutrition for the kidneys is Corn Silk.

For you to enjoy good health you need to recognize these seven channels of elimination. I plead with you to understand.

For you to be successful in your Weight loss and Detoxification journey; you need to familiarize yourself with these seven channels of removal and do everything possible to ensure they are working properly.

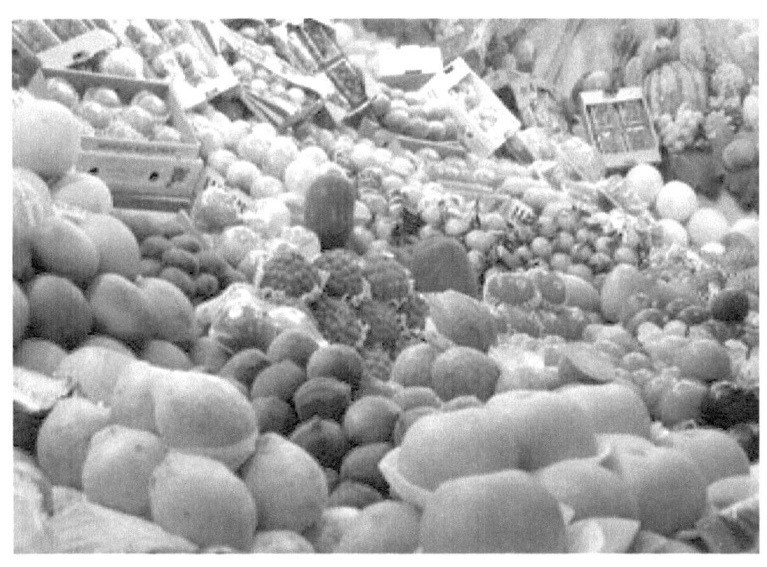

Detox Diets for weight reduction - Their risks and advantages.

Detox diets for weight reduction, just like the lemonade eating regimen recipe, have turn out to be very famous nowadays. This isn't always a terrible issue. Detoxifying can be an important aspect in shedding weight. The trouble lies in the truth that marketers have promoted them as a one prevent way to weight reduction without citing their risky outcomes and how to prevent them. While it is straight forward to lose several pounds within the first week, what dieters don't know is that approximately the detox method can purpose them to gain extra weight inside three weeks because of a false impression surrounding the metabolic technique. possibly extra startling is the truth that some of the diets do no longer properly account for electrolyte substitute that can cause the dieter to revel in some of side consequences along with muscle spasms, convulsions, abnormal heart beat, and fatigue.

Detox diets for weight reduction perform on the sound major that a build up of heavy metals, meals components, and sever different pollution in fats cells, impair the liver's capability to effectively technique fats out of the body because it's far too busy processing these pollution. With the aid of flushing that pollution out, you are ensuring that your body is burning fat and metabolizing energy in the maximum efficient manner.

The flushing method is commonly carried out through the use of a natural stool softener, observed with the aid of a natural laxative formulation.

Many of those formulas are based totally on a natural juice cleanse, the most famous being the lemonade weight-reduction plan recipe.

Alas, while the flush does expel pollution from your body, it additionally expels an entire host of minerals which might be collectively called electrolytes.

These minerals are wanted by the body to maintain fundamental nerve and muscle functions. Failure to replace those minerals can lead to decreased motor characteristic or even death in intense cases. Many juices cleanse recipes no longer name for the addition of any ingredient to correct this mineral imbalance.

In one lemonade weight-reduction plan recipe, the lively ingredients are lemon juice, cayenne pepper, and maple syrup, none of that are good enough for addressing loss of electrolytes. Earlier than the usage of the lemonade weight-reduction plan recipe, or one similar, it is vital that a dieter educate themselves on the way to upload these lacking minerals to the recipe.

Dieters should also put together themselves for the paradoxical situation that the primary pounds misplaced are the very best, and that the more weight you lose, the more difficult it will become to lose more. The purpose is that opposite to famous opinion, obese humans commonly have faster metabolisms.
This is due to the fact larger bodies require more

calories to characteristic and therefore, they should metabolize ingredients into energy at a faster rate. While a heavy character begins a food plan and restricts calorie intake, they burn those energy with a quicker metabolic price. Yet once they have misplaced some kilos and their metabolism begins to slow, they burn future calories at that slower metabolic charge which makes the technique much less efficient and tougher. This is why Detox diets for weight loss are so powerful inside the first week; however fail to supply consequences long term. Instead of preventing this uphill conflict that maximum dieters discover themselves in, the solution is to use a Detox weight loss plan as only the first step in a larger diet regime. The Detox must be observed by using a healthy diet weight-reduction plan this is metabolically adaptive to make sure that the dieter is always burning calories as efficaciously as viable and now not preventing in opposition to their personal body.

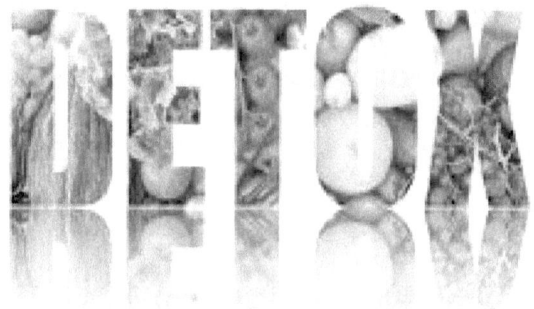

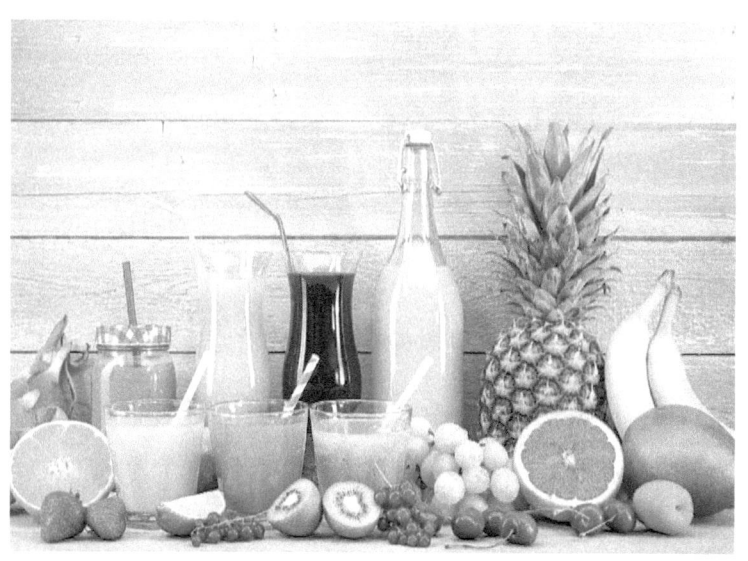

Detox Diet to pass Marijuana tests

Are you about to get examined for marijuana?

The best way to pass a Drug test for Marijuana:

Generally testing takes place for those applying for brand new jobs or people who work in industries in which an existing employer has a random drug test policy.

What type of drug test am I getting?

First you want to figure out what sort of drug check you will get. The most popular type of drug tests performed is a urinalysis which checks for the presence of marijuana inside your urine.

Urinalysis tests account for about seventy five% of drug tests; hair analysis and blood tests make up for the other 24 % with approximately 1% of tests is saliva based.

Some employers use third party drug testing labs to carry out drug tests. As the test taker, you're furnished with the address, scheduled time to visit and carry out the tests. Drug checks are usually accomplished by lab technician. Smaller employers purchase check kits and self-administer the test. This eBook will take a look at how to successfully carry out most common drug test: urinalysis, or a urine check.

How do I flush my body system of marijuana to pass a drug test?

First you have to understand that Marijuana cannot be cleaned from your system with the aid of ANY OF these items: cranberry juice, golden seal, niacin, bleach, vinegar, surejell, ginger root tea, certa or creatine capsules.

These are non effective remedies most of them have never worked and have continued to spread on-line as false truths. Any of the above stated methods has not pass present day employment drug tests.

Here's what you could DO to pass Marijuana drug test:

Trusted way to cleanse your body of Marijuana pass a drug test?

This procedure takes an estimated 30 Days based on the level of your body toxin's metabolism and your complete health.

1. Drink plenty of Water: Hydrate your body is certainly one of the key methods to flush marijuana out of your body, it isn't always a magic solution. Drinking plenty of water will allow the body properly hydrated and healthy that's one of the most essential things to do when you want to pass marijuana test to apply for your new Job.

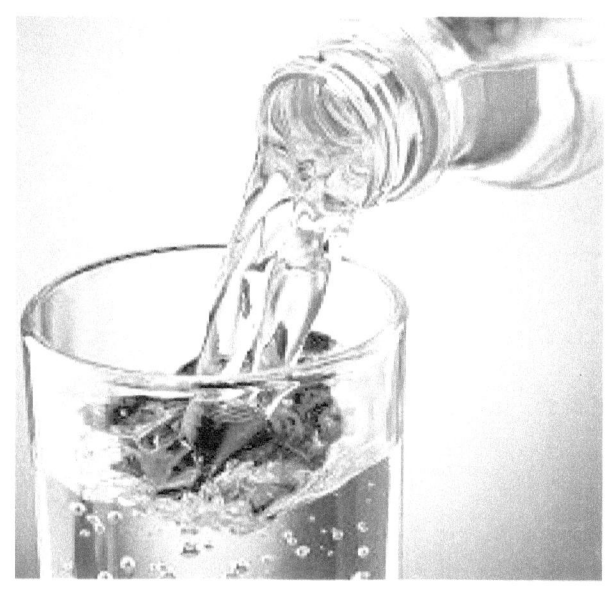

2.   Get your body exercise:
Marijuana is fat soluble and
may be saved within the fat
cells of your body, the extra
body fat you have the longer
it's going to take to detox.
The greatest way to exercise

is to use a combination of weight lifting and cardio type system like swimming or going for walks a good way to burn fats and help accelerate the metabolism.

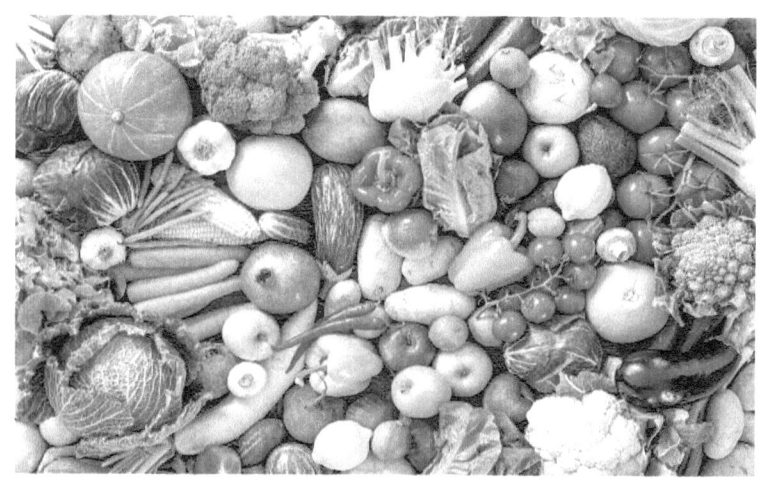

3. Eat Your Leafy greens vegetables like kale, broccoli, spinach, and chard are splendid high in vitamins and minerals like iron. These greens contain vital nutrients needed for speeding up the body metabolism.

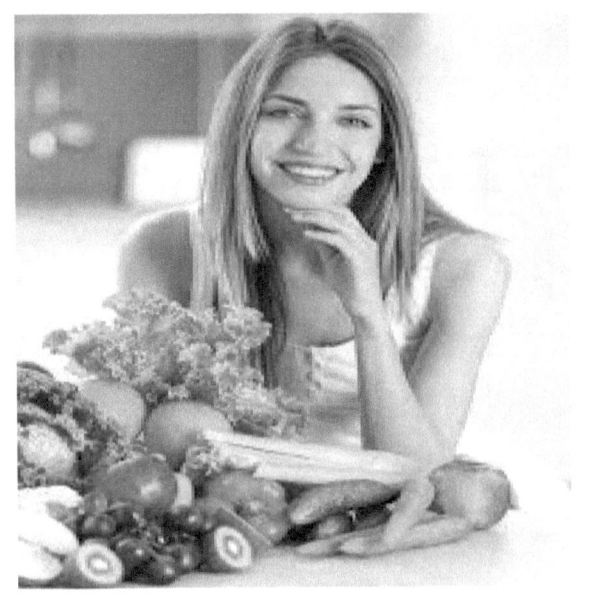

4. Drink Lemon Juice: The level of vitamin C in lemon is quite high, they are vital electrolyte and also a superb way to detox THC naturally. It is good for you to get fresh and clean lemons from the grocery store because

artificial juice from store will not have the same potency as fresh sparkling squeezed lemons.

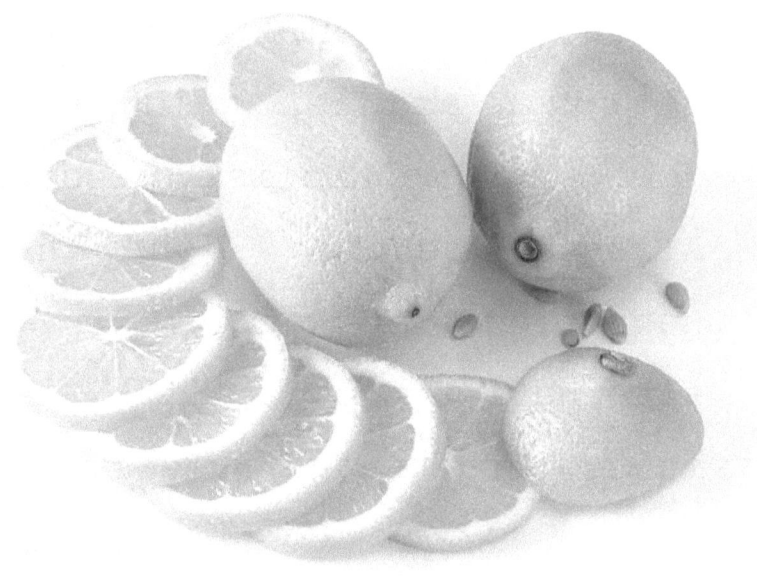

5. Avoid junk food and red meat:

Junk meals, fast meals hamburgers (yummy!) are

unhealthy generally and when it comes to detoxing marijuana they cannot help. This kind of food contains excess sodium which leads to water retention, high level of sugar and fat which slows down the metabolism process. Always settle for high nutritious food as alternative foods like lean meats, fruits and greens.

6. Adjust your type of Tea: There are several varieties of tea that helps detoxify the body of marijuana

naturally. E.g. Dandelion tea do enable the liver to flush away toxins from the body. Also Green Tea is an excellent way to boost up the because of the high levels of antioxidants, electrolytes and vitamin-C.

Any tea that has a small amount of caffeine will increase your metabolism and burn extra fats.

7. Try to eat healthy and wholesome Fiber:

Good source of healthful fiber can be in form of grains, whole wheat that has not been enriched, and legumes which consist of peas, peanuts, lentils, soy, and beans. These provide healthful nutrients needed for healthy body detoxification.

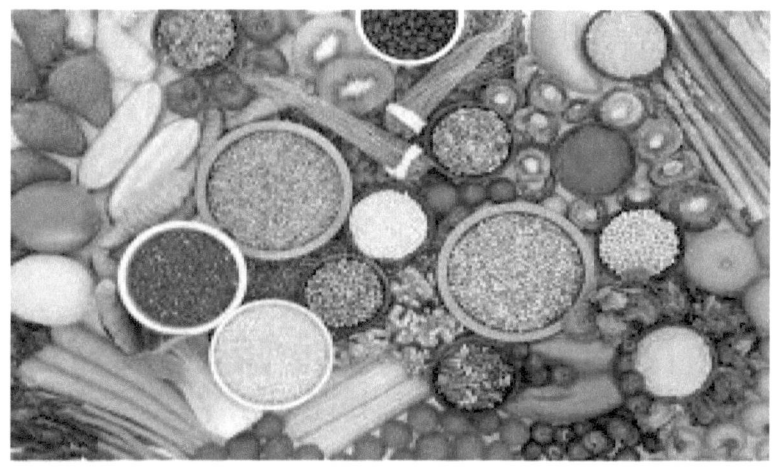

8. Try Hard to Abstain from Marijuana while Detoxing is

on-going – the usage of marijuana at some stage in your cleanse will re-deposit THC into your body and make you dirty again. The natural cleansing procedure will restart again begin from scratch when you re-introduce toxins into your body.

10. Do home test of your self-

Get a home test kit at your local drug keep or online to confirm you're completely free from marijuana.

Most popular Questions and solutions on the way to pass marijuana Drug test:

How long does it takes for marijuana to stay in to your body system?

Research endorse that marijuana can be cleansed naturally from your body through herbal detoxification, weight loss plan and workout in approximately 30 days as long as you are in suitable health and decent shape. Don't forget, you need to abstain from using marijuana during this period completely.

In excessive cases, Marijuana can stay in your blood and urine for as much as sixteen weeks depending on your toxin levels and body fat. If you weigh over two hundred kilos or have a high body fats percent, it can take this long to be clean through natural cleansing, weight loss plan and exercise.

Marijuana can stay inside your hair for 6-365 days but laboratory tests only look out for the last 90 days of hair grow. Laboratories can't test your head or body hair if your hair is pretty short. Marijuana tests have become more popular with better paying jobs and bigger employers.

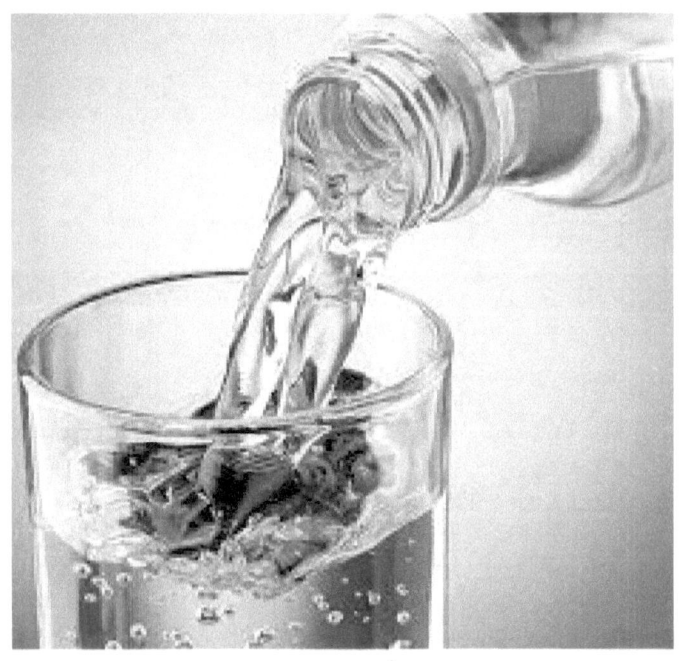

Recommended Detox Diet Resources

One week diet

Lean Belly Breakthrough

Fat Decimator System

Conclusion

The role that Detoxification plays in our diet and weight loss cannot be over emphasize therefore we need to take cognizance of our health and applied if not all parts of the strategies discussed in this book to achieve natural and healthy detox-cleansing for the benefits of our inner body system.

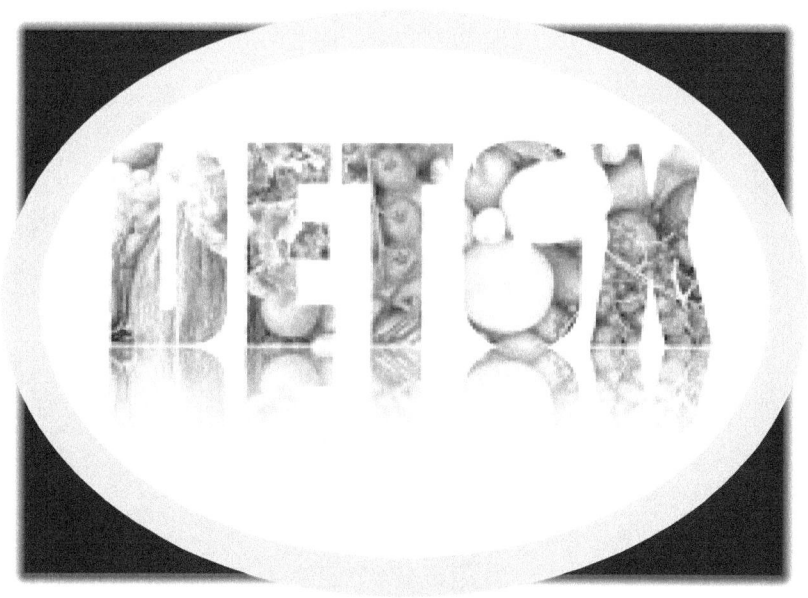

www.ingramcontent.com/pod-product-compliance
Lightning Source LLC
Chambersburg PA
CBHW021604280526

45784CB00001BA/498